Purpose-Driven Parenting

Utilizing mindfulness, positive reinforcement, and emotional intelligence to foster discipline and connection in toddlers through holistic approaches.

Michele L. Valdez

Introducing the exclusive and captivating world of Michele L. Valdez. Immerse yourself in the timeless elegance and creativity that defines our brand. Experience the unparalleled craftsmanship and attention to detail that sets us apart. Discover the essence of sophistication and style with our exquisite collection. Copyright © 2024 Michele L. Valdez

Table of Contents

PURPOSE-DRIVEN PARENTING 1

PREFACE 4

INTRODUCTION 8

CHAPTER 1..10

    DISCOVER THE ESSENTIAL GUIDE TO PARENTING 10

    UNLOCK THE SECRETS TO ENHANCING YOUR CHILD'S BEHAVIOR...................15

CHAPTER 2..25

    DISCOVER THE ART OF DELIGHTING IN PARENTHOOD 25

CHAPTER 3..32

    DISCOVER THE TOP CONCERNS EVERY PARENT OF TODDLERS SHOULD KNOW 32

CHAPTER 4..37

    DISCOVER THE ULTIMATE GUIDE TO SUCCESSFULLY NURTURING A TODDLER..................37

CHAPTER 5..45

    THE NINE GUIDELINES FOR SELF-CONTROL IN TODDLERS 45

CHAPTER 6..51

    EFFECTIVE CHILD SELF-DISCIPLINE METHODS 51

ACKNOWLEDGEMENTS..60

Preface

Are you weary of constantly fighting to keep your child under control and foster a good relationship with them? Do outbursts and confrontations about authority make you feel helpless and disengaged? It's time to set off on a life-changing adventure towards mindful toddler discipline. This journey will alter your perspective on your child's conduct as well as how you parent.

Parenting has become a difficult balancing act in our fast-paced society, particularly when it comes to navigating the rough seas of toddlerhood. However, what if I told you about a novel method of disciplining toddlers that doesn't use force or punishment? What if you could manage your child's conduct and at the same time develop a stronger bond with them?

The introduction to "Purpose-Driven Parenting: Utilizing Mindfulness, Positive Reinforcement, and Emotional Intelligence to Foster Discipline and Connection in Toddlers through Holistic Approaches."

This ground-breaking book offers a road map for realizing the full potential of your parenting experience, not just another parenting manual. "Mindful Toddler Discipline" presents a novel approach to discipline that enables parents to appreciate the present moment and develop genuine connections with their children by drawing on the concepts of mindfulness and neuroscience.

What, nevertheless, makes this book unique from the others? It's the application of mindfulness techniques to routine interactions, like as bedtime, playtime, and mealtimes. With hands-on activities, guided meditations, and examples from everyday life, you will discover how to:

Develop Presence: Learn how to give your child your whole attention even when things are chaotic. In your parenting journey, learn to let go of distractions and embrace the power of focused awareness.

Handle Difficulties with Grace: Acquire an understanding of the fundamental reasons behind your child's actions and develop empathy and compassion for them. Embrace peaceful resolutions and bid adieu to power struggles.

Develop Resilience: Give your kids the fundamental life skills they need, such as self-awareness, emotional control, and empathy. Encourage them to develop a sense of confidence and security that will last long after they are toddlers.

Don't, however, just believe what we say. See what some of our earliest readers thought about this:

"As a father, this book has completely changed my life. It's more important to comprehend my child's behavior deeply than to try to manage it. Never before have I felt closer to my toddler." - **Sarah, a dual-mother**

"As a working mother, I value the useful advice and simple workouts that I can incorporate into my everyday schedule. Our family's dynamic has improved as a result of mindful parenting." - **Emily, a working mother**

Are you prepared to set off on a path of introspection and change? Come along as we reimagine what it means to be mindfully and lovingly disciplined. In your home, bid dissatisfaction by and welcome to harmony.

I applaud you for starting your journey toward purpose-driven parenting by ordering your copy today!

But there's still more! In addition, as a unique extra, you'll have access to premium online tools like worksheets, guided meditations, and a community of like-minded parents. Additionally, keep an eye out for the author's upcoming webinars and workshops, where you may delve deeper into the concepts of mindful parenting.

Don't allow another day to pass you by feeling helpless and disengaged. It's time to get your happiness and self-assurance back as a parent. Get the most out of your parenting abilities by utilizing "Purpose-Driven Parenting."

Introduction

The groundbreaking book "Purpose-Driven Parenting," written by renowned author Michelle L. Valdez, redefines contemporary parenting. Families are overloaded with distractions in the digital era, so it's critical that we rediscover our basic beliefs. This ground-breaking book presents a revolutionary parenting philosophy that goes beyond simple discipline and emphasizes creating a purpose for every part of family life.

Michele L. Valdez enables parents to foster meaningful connections with their children and develop a sense of purpose from an early age by providing incisive insights and useful advice. Through the development of empathy, resilience, creativity, and ambition, "Purpose-Driven Parenting" gives you the tools to create motivated, caring people who are ready to change the world.

This book provides a road map for consciously and gracefully negotiating the challenges of contemporary parenthood, drawing on the most recent findings in child psychology and personal development research. Learn how to build a nurturing environment, prioritize family values, and set realistic goals so that kids can grow up to be emotionally, intellectually, and socially successful.

"Purpose-Driven Parenting" offers priceless insights and doable solutions for every step of your child's journey, whether you're navigating the tumultuous adolescent years or the struggles of toddlerhood. Bid adieu to autopilot parenting and welcome a more purpose-driven, fulfilling style of parenting that will benefit your family for years to come.

This is the book you've been looking for if you're ready to take off on a transforming parenting adventure full of passion, purpose, and deep relationships. Join the innumerable families throughout the globe that have experienced incredible changes in their relationships and the lives of their children as a result of embracing the power of purpose-driven parenting. It's time to take back your position as a parent with a purpose and help create a better future for future generations.

Chapter 1

Discover the Essential Guide to Parenting

Unlock the secrets of seamlessly navigating the journey of your child's growth, from precious infant to curious toddler. Mastering this art is an essential skill for parents, guardians, and caregivers alike.

Experience the remarkable journey of a child's growth as it unfolds in various areas of development:

- Experience the remarkable journey of physical development as your child's size increases and they grow into their full potential.

- Introducing the extraordinary primary movement skills: Mastering the art of controlling colossal moving toys. With this newfound ability, children can effortlessly stroll, operate, jump, rise, and walk with utmost grace and precision.

- Introducing Vision: Unlock the power to observe with precision and effortlessly comprehend the world around you.

- Unlock the power of hearing and speech: Experience the extraordinary ability to effortlessly hear, absorb vital information, seamlessly process it with utmost clarity, and effortlessly interpret the world around you. Discover the remarkable capability to effortlessly comprehend and harness the power of words, enabling you to effortlessly connect and communicate with unparalleled effectiveness.

- Introducing Sociable: Unlock the power to effortlessly connect with people all around the globe.

- Discover the power of visual representation with graphs to define intervals of advancement. But don't forget, improvement is a continuous journey and what may appear as 'abnormal' could simply be a unique path to growth.

- Introducing the One-Year-Old: A Milestone Worth Celebrating!

- Discover the incredible abilities that a one-year-old

child can possess:

- Unlock your full potential with our cutting-edge physical and motion skills training. Elevate your performance to new heights and achieve unparalleled success.

- Discover the astonishing body mass of an average one-year-old toddler.

- Experience the ultimate convenience with our delivery service that triples the weight of your order. No more worrying about multiple trips or heavy lifting - we've got you covered!

- Experience exponential growth, reaching an impressive 50% increase above the initial delivery height.

- Introducing our incredible teeth growth formula! Experience the amazing transformation of growing 1 - 8 teeth with ease.

- Introducing the revolutionary "Draw to Stand"! Experience the ultimate convenience and efficiency with our innovative product. Say goodbye to the hassle of bending down and struggling to reach your items. With "Draw to Stand," everything is within your grasp. Elev

- Experience the freedom to walk, with or without assistance.

- Experience the ultimate in relaxation with our revolutionary Sit Back Without Help chair. Say goodbye to discomfort and hello to pure bliss as you sink into the plush cushions and let the chair do all the work. Whether you're reading a book, watching a movie, or simply unwinding after a long

- Experience the exhilarating sound of two blocks colliding!

- Experience the joy of effortlessly flipping through the pages of a book, as if each page is eagerly vying for your attention. With a simple flick, multiple pages come alive, inviting you to embark on a captivating journey.

- Experience the incredible dexterity of a pincer grasp.

- Experience the rejuvenating power of a full 8-10 hours of restful sleep at night, complemented by invigorating power naps throughout the day.

- Experience the extraordinary benefits of sensory and cognitive advancement.

- Discover the art of dining with utmost independence.

- Chase after an effortlessly gliding object.

- Introducing our revolutionary feature: the ability to respond to your pet's name! Say goodbye to the days of your furry friend ignoring you. With our cutting-edge technology, we've made it possible for your pet to recognize and respond to their name like never before. Experience the joy of

- Discover a vast vocabulary.

- Introducing a little one who effortlessly utters

endearing terms like "mom" and "dad" with absolute charm.

- Discover the power of mastering basic commands.

- Experience the joy of mimicking your beloved pet's noises.

- Introducing our revolutionary feature: Title-to-Item Connection!

- Discover the power of recognizing the presence of products, even when they remain unseen.

Unlock the Secrets to Enhancing Your Child's Behavior

Unlock the secret to nurturing well-rounded children by embracing the power of proper parenting. Small kids, with their endearing yet sometimes challenging behaviors, require our keen observation, attentive listening, and timely assistance. Discover the transformative impact of implementing these essential parenting ideas.

Discover the joys and challenges of connecting with

children, making life an exhilarating journey. Discover the secret to achieving perfect harmony with your little ones. While we strive for fairness, it's important to remember that children may not always keep up with our pace. Their boundless needs and desires often lead to negotiation and discontent. Experience the inevitable outcome of tantrums and misbehaviors.

Transform your child into a well-behaved superstar with the power of superior guidance and unwavering love:

- Discover the Ultimate Guide to Enhancing Your Child's Behavior with These Invaluable Suggestions!

- Discover the secrets to success with these invaluable tips.

- Express your emotions in style.

Experience the power of love as you shower your child with affection that surpasses any form of punishment. Embrace, caress, and radiate a warm and friendly attitude to instill in your children a deep sense of your unwavering love and appreciation. Similarly, showering them with kind words, genuine compliments, and undivided attention can serve as powerful catalysts to inspire and uplift their spirits.

Introducing: Prioritize Guidelines - Your Ultimate Solution!

Revamp your approach to parenting by ditching the overwhelming barrage of rules and principles that only serve to ignite your child's anger. Instead, focus on prioritizing the ones that safeguard their well-being and safety. And don't forget to sprinkle in some valuable tips to help shape their future. Transform your home into a safe haven for your little one by implementing childproofing measures and eliminating any potential hazards.

Put an end to those dreaded tantrums!

Discover the secret to managing your child's temper tantrums with ease. Don't just aim to prevent them, but significantly reduce their frequency. Discover the true power and timing of your child's tantrums with these essential tips:

Discover the true potential of your child: Unlock the secret to well-behaved children by ensuring they fully comprehend your every request. Don't let misbehavior be a barrier - make sure your kid understands exactly what you're asking for.

Discover the art of evaluating and fine-tuning your rules and principles. Instead of simply instructing others to cease striking, why not provide them with valuable suggestions on how to achieve a different outcome?

Discover the power of 'NO' as a sign of advancement: Discover the power of positive persuasion when your child utters the word "no." Instead of overreacting, why not take a different approach? Engage in a gentle yet persuasive manner that encourages them to reconsider and give it another try. Discover the secret to transforming your work into a thrilling adventure with the power of games! Unlock your child's potential by transforming their tasks into enjoyable experiences. When you infuse work with a sense of fun, you'll be amazed at how effortlessly they follow your lead.

Choose your battles wisely: Unlock the potential of your child by embracing the power of 'YES'. When you say 'NO' to every opportunity, you risk dampening their spirits and stifling their growth. Choose to inspire and motivate your little one by being open to new experiences and possibilities. Unlock the power of discernment by keenly observing the perfect moments to confidently say YES.

Introducing a world of possibilities: Ignite your child's sense of independence by empowering them to choose their own pajamas or bedtime story.

Discover the secret to a harmonious environment by steering clear of circumstances that have the potential to ignite disappointment or unleash tantrums: Introducing the perfect solution: avoid the mistake of gifting your child toys that are beyond their developmental stage. Discover the art of balancing your child's activities with much-needed rest. Determine whether it's time for play or a moment of relaxation, and avoid prolonged outings.

Discover the importance of acknowledging that children need rest when they are feeling fatigued, hungry, unwell, or in an unfamiliar setting.

Experience the transformative power of our program: Introducing a well-crafted day-to-day routine, ensuring your child is always in the know and prepared for what lies ahead.

Ignite the power of effective communication: Discover the perfect solution to encourage your child to effectively communicate their emotions. Discover the secret to effective communication with your child. Unlock a world of possibilities by introducing them to the captivating world of baby sign vocabulary. Don't let your child's quiet nature hold them back - empower them to express themselves confidently and avoid any potential disappointment. Embrace the power of baby sign vocabulary today!

Be a trendsetter: Unlock the incredible power of observation in children as they effortlessly grasp new skills by simply watching their parents in action.

Introducing the ultimate method to instill proper behavior in your child: by setting a shining example for them to witness firsthand.

Experience the power of enforce effects: Introducing a scenario where even with your utmost dedication, your child may inadvertently stray from the guidelines. Discover the power of overlooking minor displays of anger, such as when a young one unleashes strikes, kicks, or screams for an extended duration. Instead, embrace a careful approach to assisting children with any challenges they may be facing. Discover the power of alternative child-rearing techniques that will effortlessly inspire your little one to collaborate.

Discover the Ultimate Guide to Child Rearing Tips: Unleash the Power of Organic Consequences!

Unlock the power of teaching your child about the impact of their actions, all while ensuring their safety. Introducing a brilliant solution: imagine a world where your child's toys remain intact, unharmed by accidental mishaps. Picture this: if your little one happens to throw and break a toy, they won't have access to that particular gadget anymore, preventing any further instances of damage. Say goodbye to repetitive repairs and hello to a worry-free playtime experience!

Introducing: Reasonable Consequences

Ensure that your child has all the necessary supplies for their activities, and emphasize the importance of handling their play toys with care. Remind them that if they are not careful, the toys may need to be temporarily put away. Empower your child with unwavering support, going above and beyond when needed. Discover the power of effective communication with your child. Ensure they understand the importance of cooperation by clearly explaining the consequences.

Unleash the Power of Freedom

Discover the secret to managing your child's misbehavior with ease. Take control by strategically removing any triggers that may be fueling their unruly behavior. Whether it's their beloved toy or an object linked to their misdeeds, simply eliminate it from their grasp and watch as harmony is restored.

Experience the ultimate break with our exclusive "Time-out" package.

Experience the power of effective parenting when your child misbehaves. Take a moment to connect with them on their level, delivering a calm and concise explanation as to why their behavior is less than desirable. Experience the transformative power of nature by taking your child to a carefully chosen outdoor location. Find solace in a serene and uninterrupted environment, away from the hustle and bustle of daily life, where your child can truly thrive. Experience the power of enforcing a time-out until your child is fully relaxed and able to focus solely on you. Ensure your child of unwavering support, every step of the way.

Choose your consequences wisely and stick to them with unwavering consistency.

Experience peace of mind knowing that every responsible adult who plays a role in your child's life is fully committed to following these essential guidelines and discipline recommendations.

Introducing a gentle reminder to be mindful when it comes to evaluating your child's behavior. Discover the compassionate and effective approach to parenting that avoids the harmful methods of spanking, slapping, and shouting. Embrace a nurturing and respectful environment for your young child.

C h a p t e r 2

Discover the Art of Delighting in Parenthood

Experience the triumph over sleepless nights and endless feeding cycles of the newborn stage. Cherish the precious moments of cuddling adorable baby cheeks and witnessing every new milestone. But alas, that chapter of life has come to a close.

Discover the exhilarating journey of parenting young kids, where every day brings a thrilling adventure. Brace yourself for a world filled with endless surprises and heartwarming moments, as children are notorious for their unpredictable antics. From their mischievous pranks to their innocent curiosity, be prepared to embark on a remarkable voyage like no other.

Unlock the power of communication with them - although their preferred phrase is undoubtedly "no."

Experience the freedom of effortless movement. Picture this: they gracefully stroll, but beware, they may also attempt to elude you in parking lots.

Discover the incredible impartiality that emerges when they are presented with something between the ages of 2 and 4. It's a phenomenon that never fails to amaze!

Discover the ultimate guide to cultivating a culture of respect in children and pre-schoolers towards their beloved parents or caregivers. Discover the utmost importance of nurturing your bond with your child, a connection that is not only significant but also vital for their well-being. Embrace the opportunity to savor this extended period of growth and development, as you navigate the journey of parenthood.

Discover the Ultimate Guide to Nurturing a Young Mind

Are you a parent looking to navigate the challenging world of discipline? It's crucial to understand that skipping the initial discipline stage can hinder your toddler's development of self-discipline. Don't let parenting become a headache - let's explore the importance of this crucial step together.

Prepare yourself for an exhilarating journey filled with endless power challenges, captivatingly intense and delightfully eccentric behavior, and truly legendary meltdowns that will leave you in awe.

Discover the transformative power of positive parenting with our unique approach. Immerse yourself in this transformative ideology that effortlessly allows you to unwind and forge deep connections with these remarkable children, even in the face of their occasional misbehavior. Discover how it empowers you to provide unwavering support to help them navigate through psychological challenges, while imparting invaluable life lessons using the most reliable and effective techniques available.

Discover the transformative power of this unique parenting approach that effortlessly enhances your child's behavior. Unlock the secret to effectively managing those challenging moments when your little one acts out. Remember to consider their age, developmental stage, and brain maturity for optimal results. Discover the moment when you become aware that your child is experiencing confusion in a specific situation and is in desperate need of some well-deserved rest.

Experience the power of our carefully crafted stages, each one delivering impactful solutions and strategies that truly work. Our expert team ensures that every solution we provide leaves you feeling relaxed and in complete control. Discover the difference today.

Introducing the ultimate guide to effectively disciplining young kids: a must-read for all parents! First and foremost, let's delve into the true essence of "self-discipline" and "consequence."

Introducing "Punishment/Consequence" - a revolutionary approach to instilling discipline in your child. Our carefully crafted penalties are designed to evoke a sense of profound discomfort, ensuring effective instruction and long-lasting results. Introducing "Self-discipline" - the ultimate tool to guide your child towards a more effective approach in managing challenges, without the need for punishment.

Discover the power of a seemingly modest collection of words that can have a profound impact on your interactions with your child. Discover a new approach to training that avoids the pitfalls of insults and punishment. By reframing your perspective, you can prevent labeling your child as "bad," "misbehaving," or "bratty." Discover the remarkable truth: they can effortlessly transcend the need to "escape punishment for their misdeeds" or simply learn invaluable life lessons through the power of discipline.

Unfortunately, this endeavor will not cultivate a harmonious and fulfilling connection, leaving you with a less than desirable experience in the realm of parenthood.

Discover the remarkable transformation that occurs when you observe your child after they have experienced the consequences of their actions. Prepare to be moved by a profound sense of compassion. Discover the secrets to empowering and uplifting those around you who may find it challenging to respond to sympathy. Unlock the keys to providing encouragement and unwavering support.

Introducing a whole new level of "discipline" that will revolutionize your child's development. Prepare to witness the extraordinary power of nurturing their psychological intelligence, boosting problem-solving skills, fostering empathy towards others, and cultivating a strong, healthy bond between you and your little one.

Discover the Essential Precautions to Take Before Dismissing Children

Unleash the Power of Calm: Taming Child Meltdowns and Tantrums

Unleash the full potential of your child's problem-solving skills with these powerful actions. Before jumping in to correct or offer a better solution, try these strategies:

Introducing the unrivaled masters of tantrums - youngsters! Witness their unparalleled expertise in the art of throwing fits like no other. Brace yourself for a spectacle of epic proportions! Prepare for an immersive and intense experience that frequently leaves parents feeling overwhelmed, surprised, and even ashamed.

Experience the joy of typical tantrums during the magical toddler and preschooler years. Discover the challenge of understanding every aspect of the toddler all at once.

Discover the power of the ethical child-rearing principle and unlock a world of calm and harmony for you and your child. Say goodbye to tantrums and meltdowns that disrupt your day, and embrace a more peaceful and joyful parenting experience.

Chapter 3

Discover the Top Concerns Every Parent of Toddlers Should Know

Are you exhausted and frustrated by the challenges your child faces, leaving you feeling drained and unable to provide the support they need?

Discover the secrets to a truly delightful parenting journey with these foolproof tips.

Discover the incredible responsibility that parents bear when it comes to nurturing their child's development. It's not just about self-discipline, as numerous other challenges arise unexpectedly along the way. Discover the silver lining: the vast majority of problems are anything but unique. Discover the incredible journey of personal growth that awaits every child.

Discover the power of utilizing this incredible tool to enhance your reaction when these challenging issues arise. Keep in mind that every child is unique, so be prepared for individual differences. Are you a seasoned pro when it comes to training your child? That's impressive! However, it's always important to keep an eye out for anything out of the ordinary or concerning. Don't hesitate to reach out to a trusted physician or mental wellness provider for guidance and support. After all, your child's well-being is of the utmost importance.

Introducing: The Ultimate Guide to Nurturing Toddlers through Sibling Competition and Rivalry!

- Embarking on the journey of parenting a toddler is no easy feat. But when you throw several other children into the mix, you're faced with a whole new set of challenges to conquer.

- Discover the power of nurturing your child's interpersonal skills. Rather than expecting them to effortlessly adapt, empower them with your unwavering support as they navigate the complexities of sharing toys, embracing change, and engaging in healthy arguments without causing harm to their peers.

Discover the extraordinary advice and innovative

approaches for parenting children that are not only theoretically excellent, but also have the power to transform your parenting journey. However, without the essential skill of anger management, these strategies may seem insurmountable.

Discover the secret to raising well-behaved children without ever raising your voice.

Discover the secret to maintaining your composure while still ensuring the safety of your children. Instead of resorting to yelling, unleash your best performance as a parent. We understand that there may be moments when you feel overwhelmed, uncertain, or concerned about what others think. But fear not, for we have the solution to help you avoid any potential harm and preserve your child's well-being.

Escape the confines of frustration and discover a refreshing way to free your mind from the chaos of yelling. Discover the invaluable tips I have meticulously outlined for you. Choose from a selection of cutting-edge strategies that will empower you to persevere with unwavering determination and maintain an unwavering sense of optimism.

Discover the secret to transforming from an unaggressive parent to a confident one, even in those challenging moments when you find yourself raising your voice at your children.

Discover the moments when your child will rely on you to rise to the occasion, but remember, it shouldn't be a constant occurrence.

Unlock Your Full Parenting Potential with Parent Coaching!

Discover the joys and challenges of raising small kids and pre-schoolers. While it may seem like a problem at times, it can also be a rewarding and fulfilling experience. Embrace the journey, even when it feels isolating and complicated. Discover the power of a single Google search, where a world of knowledge awaits at your fingertips. While your friends may have their own unique perspectives on raising a child, it's important to remember that their advice may not always align with your specific parenting needs.

Don't go it alone in the world of parenting - you deserve some much-needed support. Discover the incredible benefits of obtaining parenting guidance from books! With a success rate of over 70%, this safe and reliable method provides you with sound advice that is both non-judgmental and effective. By following a proven training pattern, you can ensure a fantastic experience for both you and your child.

Feeling overwhelmed by everything that has been mentioned? Don't worry, if you're unsure of where to begin, there's no need to panic. Unlock the possibilities that lie before us by embracing the notion that there is always a path to success. Only when we wholeheartedly commit ourselves to meeting the demands it presents can we truly achieve greatness.

Chapter 4

Discover the Ultimate Guide to Successfully Nurturing a Toddler

Discover the transformative power of our carefully curated methodologies for raising your child. By incorporating these proven techniques into your parenting journey, you can unlock a world of possibilities and make an extraordinary impact on your child's development.

Be a leader in your own right:

Feel the urge to take control when things seem uncontrollable? It's only natural. However, there are several other things that are beyond our control. Discover the secret to harmonious relationships with your child. By embracing a more mindful approach to parenting, you can avoid the common pitfalls of power struggles. Say goodbye to unnecessary conflicts and hello to a peaceful and loving connection with your little one. Discover the power to shape your personal behavior and unlock the potential for your child to follow in your footsteps. Experience the power of collaboration and strengthen the bond with your child by becoming true partners. Working together as a team, you'll unlock a world of positive effects through deep connection and seamless cooperation.

Embrace the Power of Positivity: Have you ever been told that "Whatever you focus on, grows?" Experience the transformative power of this unique perspective, as it effortlessly shapes your thoughts, stirs your emotions, and ignites your deepest feelings. Unlock your child's potential by empowering them with the knowledge of their own capabilities. Take a moment to acknowledge and celebrate their achievements, fueling their motivation to excel even further. Experience the incredible benefits that come with unwavering dedication. Empower your child and enhance the senses of everyone involved. Discover a world of strength and growth.

Unlock the power of connection:

Discover the incredible potential of small children as

they embark on their journey towards independence. While they may possess remarkable abilities from the start, they continue to rely on us for emotional support and guidance. Discover the undeniable importance of relationships during the crucial stage of toddlerhood. Discover the power of connecting with your child in the midst of challenging circumstances, as it can greatly contribute to their overall psychological well-being and balance. Experience the power of a deep connection as it unlocks the potential for a child to learn, grow, and thrive.

Unlock your full potential with our revolutionary approach to focus and study. Say goodbye to distractions and hello to laser-like concentration. Experience the power of our proven techniques and watch your productivity soar. Don't just study

Discover the innate human tendency to appreciate aesthetics. Discover the remarkable truth that even though parents may be wise and experienced, it does not mean they should underestimate the importance of a toddler's emotions, feelings, and thoughts. Discover the foolproof method to effortlessly capture a child's attention: simply ignore them.

Experience a wide range of emotions and feelings, as they are all part of the human experience. But remember, not all actions are created equal. Choose wisely.

Experience the full spectrum of human emotions with our innate programming. Unlock the power of emotional intelligence in your child's journey towards growth and development. By fostering an environment where emotions and feelings are embraced, you can empower them to cultivate a positive mindset. Remember, acknowledging their emotions does not equate to endorsing any excessive or undesirable behaviors. Unlock the power of emotional intelligence in your child by guiding them to navigate their emotions with ease and clarity. Instead of suppressing their feelings, empower them to embrace and understand their emotional landscape. Discover the power of assisting others in navigating the intricate realm of expressing their deepest emotions and thoughts through impeccable conduct.

Discover the power of seeking assistance when it comes

to understanding your child's behavior. Attention is undeniably one of the most reliable tools at our disposal when it comes to effective parenting. Discover the power of seeking assistance when it comes to understanding your toddler's behavior. Uncover the hidden depths of their world. Experience the power of undivided attention, forging a deep connection that empowers you to respond thoughtfully instead of reacting impulsively when faced with disappointment.

Discover the true driving force behind the behavior, rather than simply fixating on the action at hand:

Unlock the secret to understanding your toddler's behavior - it's all about emotions, feelings, and needs! Discover the secret to transforming behavior effortlessly by shifting your focus away from the action itself. Discover the true power of directing your attention towards the principal act, the very catalyst that holds the potential to create real change. Experience the transformative power of acknowledging and addressing your emotions, feelings, and needs, as it revolutionizes your behavior.

Unlock your full potential with our cutting-edge performance solutions. Experience the power of peak performance as you tackle your main work with ease and confidence.

Experience the joy of your toddler's boundless imagination as they venture into the great outdoors. Encourage their unstructured creativity and watch as they develop a sense of autonomy and control. By embracing the outdoors, your child will not only have fun, but also acquire valuable new skills.

Unleash their curiosity and exceed their expectations: Young minds are naturally curious, eager to explore the wonders of the world. However, they require ample time to fully grasp the complexities of understanding this vast and fascinating planet. Discover the potential of those who may be facing developmental challenges, as they have a unique way of expressing themselves through their behavior.

Discover the power of uplifting others, not through insults and abuse, but by imparting the essential skills they require to thrive and exceed expectations in the future.

Experience the power of taking a breath and putting it to the ultimate test. Embrace the journey of gradual progress and unlock your true potential. Experience the exhilaration of self-recognition as you generously reward yourself with a resounding appraisal. Embrace each new day with renewed vigor and strive to unleash your utmost potential.

Experience the transformative power of change. Embrace the journey that unfolds over time, as you cultivate new habits and refine your skills. With unwavering dedication and the right support, you can unlock your true potential. Seize the potential of each day as a stepping stone towards readiness for whatever lies ahead.

Don't let any mistake bring you down. Rise above and keep pushing forward. Discover the truth: even the most devoted parents are not immune to making mistakes. Unlock the power of probability and embark on a journey of endless learning. Experience the magic of each passing minute as an irresistible opportunity to embark on a fresh new journey.

Chapter 5

The Nine Guidelines for Self-Control in Toddlers

Because of the functional relationship and tie that exists between you and your children, it is not a good idea to allow them to grow too accustomed to rules and consequences.

Offspring that do not necessarily possess gregarious traits often exhibit the typical individual trait of a survival-of-the-fittest mentality. For this reason, you should teach your child the proper and safe way to perform certain tasks.

Later on, the seeds of self-control will sprout, and the results of your labor will truly astound you. These are the instructions that you must follow:

Be prepared for tight circumstances: There are situations and moments in your life when you are more likely to act out. There's a common misconception that switching from one activity to another alerts your child, making them more prepared for advancements.

Pick your battles: Saying "no" twenty times a day will gradually make the word less meaningful. Sort activities into three categories: large, medium, and too small to use.

Stop specific things from occurring: While making your house kid-friendly, maintain your standards. Your child won't be tempted to throw everything if all of your movie collections are arranged neatly on your desk. Go ahead and eat dinner early if you are taking your entire family out; this indicates that you won't be holding them back.

Assist in keeping your claims succinct and enjoyable: Use succinct language to convey the message, such "No biting." Compared to "Chase," which sounds more like you're speaking to your dog, it is far more effective.

Refocus and divert: If your child has unrolled the entire roll of toilet paper, for example, quickly remove him or her from the restroom and shut the door.

Introduce the effects: Your children need to understand that their actions have repercussions. For example, if he/she strongly insists on choosing the pajamas to wear (which takes a long time), there won't be any time left to learn before bed.

Cause: Constantly picking up pajamas.

Effect: Learning and discovery take very little time. The following time, he or she would either let you choose their pajamas for them or choose them fast.

Don't back down to prevent conflict: Make the right choice if you decide that your child won't eat the cereal she sees on TV. You'll be happy you did later.

Prepare offers of interest in advance: Yes, your little angel will approach you whenever you're talking on the phone or preparing dinner, which is usually when your attention is diverted. For this reason, it's essential to have multiple forms of entertainment available (such as a device or a quick treat).

Focus on the behavior, not the child: it's okay to criticize a specific conduct, but you should never tell your child that they are evil.

Give your child options: She might feel that she has a voice because of this. Make sure you give him/her a lot of options.

You often find yourself yelling: Yelling is acceptable as long as you adjust the pitch of your voice. Screaming to the top of your lungs usually does nothing, but the firmness of your voice conveys the message. Recall that there was never really anything to be angry about.

Encourage your child: If you give them lots of praise for excellent behavior, they'll be more likely to behave nicely in the future and may be less likely to act out in order to obtain attention. In general, the super-ego is fertilized by positive reinforcement.

Think about acting right away: Don't wait for your child to always grasp a concept, and don't assume that they can always discipline themselves.

Think about setting an example for your child. If you are calm and not cruel, they will pick up on the hint. Additionally, anticipate that he may act similarly if you have a short fuse and are agitated. He's always keeping an eye on you.

Handle your child as an adult: You don't have to listen to a child's lengthy speech because it's possible that they won't even comprehend it. For example, don't include too many lectures; instead, forcefully instruct on how to carry out the activity the next time he or she wants to make spaghetti incorrectly.

Use time-outs: for a one-year-old, you may need to think about preventing your child from playing and not focusing on him every minute. It can be easy to communicate with him if you deny him attention.

It's a fact that toddlers under two years old will not likely curl up in a corner or inside a seat, therefore it's a great idea to let them kick and scream on the floor. Just make sure it's a safe place for the time-out.

After a while, alter your tactics: What was incredibly effective when your child was 15 weeks old is probably not going to be effective when he is two years old.

Don't spank: Refrain, even if you find yourself tempted occasionally! You'll observe a far more efficient method of conveying the information. Tell your child it's okay to work under pressure if he starts to kick or hit you, for example. Lastly, try to take a backseat if your child is really getting on your nerves. You'll have a deeper understanding of the manipulative strategies your child is employing as well as new insight on how to enhance your approach.

Tell your child again how much you adore them: That's a great approach to initiate a discussion about self-control. This lets your child know that you're willing to move forward rather than focusing on the issue. It also confirms that you place boundaries because you cherish her.

Chapter 6

Effective Child Self-discipline Methods

It can be challenging to discipline young children, so try not to get disheartened by your children's tantrums.

Early childhood educator Denise Marshall famously remarked, "What's 'bad' behavior anyway? Every time, a child's explanation and a parent's command usually diverge greatly: You ask your youngster to put a device away. They don't. You detect disobedience. They are not required to cease playing.

Experts concur that when our expectations exceed our children's capacity, they will undoubtedly "misbehave." For example, it makes no sense to expect a youngster to pay attention to a series of instructions or even to retain a rule after hearing it once.

A daycare specialist explains, "You must use straightforward language. Their minds are constantly busy. You have to say it again, or else people will not follow your instructions.

To maintain the goals in a realistic range, it helps to learn about the developmental factors influencing toddler behavior:

Social Skills

Toddlers are starting to get along with other kids at the age of 1.5. However, children need to be taught how to take criticism and accept modifications in order to play in a sociable manner. Intense behavior, like as biting, is actually rather common. It advances development. What matters is how people react.

Restraint

The majority of disobedience that adults and children alike blame on toddler behavior stems from their inability to control their urges. Even though your partner knows that throwing food—which happens to be your favorite—is not something you should do, give it a shot because you might find yourself wanting to witness her mac and cheese go from splat to bottom more than anything else.

On the other hand, a child may react strongly if their

desires and urges are denied.

psychological control

Beyond learning to control their emotions, children struggle with understanding them. They require assistance in recognizing and addressing their feelings. Utilizing your comforting embraces could be beneficial in revealing self-soothing methods.

With sympathy

Young children may be self-centered because they are just like everyone else in the world—they are just learning. They may struggle with empathy, thus they may not truly notice how other people react negatively when they are uncomfortable or disappointed. This also clarifies why a child could react improperly to the emotions of another child, such as laughing when a playmate pinches them in order to get a toy.

Understanding

When a young child doesn't even understand the repercussions of following instructions, how can they possibly follow them? It's important to remember that toddlers' language and attention spans are still developing, so you should never assume too much about what they can understand. "Parents should encourage their children even though they may already be aware of what their parents are asking for."

Your child won't give you his full attention even though he understands everything you're saying. "I have to admit, I haven't seen any kids who listen very often." They are at a level where you must remain composed.

What functions

In what precise way can someone mentor your child's behavior? Your child is modeling her conduct for you, therefore you should practice self-control techniques based on your values, age, and character. The following are the top tactics:

Provide options

Young children experiment with independence, thus it's critical to provide safe, appropriate spaces for them to express themselves. Some examples of these spaces include: Which would you prefer—the green cup or the deep glass—for your juice? "Which would you prefer—the newborn stroller or driving straight to the parking lot in your car?"

Oversee

Although it may not seem like a self-discipline technique, if you are not present to teach your child, you cannot assist him in learning acceptable behaviors. This entails advising them on the best course of action rather than jumping right into solving every issue.

Arranged goals and penalties

If children can not even comprehend the seriousness of the rules, they will not be able to follow them. Make sure your instructions and rules are clear and concise, such as "Make sure she's nodding when you talk to her" and "Establish eye-to-eye contact."

Show and explain

Young children are obvious; they almost absorb

everything that goes on around them. As a result, you must set an example for the conduct you desire. Therefore, you should make whatever alteration you want people to see first.

Gratitude

Even though young children have narrow minds, they nevertheless require praise. When your boy distributes his meal, remember to give him credit for it; it typically improves your bond. "Parents are meant to provide their children with the constant attention they require."

Refocus

When an opportunity presents itself for unusual behavior, divert their attention with something they enjoy doing. If your 2.5-year-old is upset that her older sibling won't talk to her about her new doll, suggest, "Let's get the sticker peel at the kitchen desk." Furthermore, kids at this age truly like lending a hand.

Additionally, redirection could "unstick" your child from a No-No. Get her involved in any new activity if

Grandma's music system has a magnetic effect on her.

Take out

Wherever you would take your child, parents should set up a productive, quiet space for them. Give in to his offer and gently remove him from his current location. It is a place to unwind rather than engage in activities. The couch, a stairway step, or an area surrounding the carpet with plush cushions aren't all that bad of an idea.

Think about what you do.

Talking to a small child after a misbehavior episode may sound reasonable, but it is useless when the child is a toddler.

Express regret

If you don't apologize after doing something wrong, it can hurt a young child.

"No, no, very little no, no..."

It is best to teach children the right and wrong things to do. Try, as soon as you can, to convey your point clearly and quietly rather than by "yelling NO."

Set clear objectives.

Make sure your instructions are clear and audible to them: "I'll set those glasses aside if you splash water through the tub again."

If you explain to older toddlers why splashing water on the floor is often dangerous, they may react. Most of us could fall because of it.

Give choices

"Which would you prefer—putting water in your cup or flask?" Giving them options indicates that we are guiding them because they might become lost in an activity.

Take out

If she keeps splashing, take her out of the tub and give her an explanation such as, "You're stubborn, so I have to take you out of the tub."

Repercussions

As she watches you mop up the spilled water, point out the outcomes of her actions by saying, "Spilled water needs to be cleaned up because someone could slip and get hurt."

Acknowledgements

Behold the magnificent triumph of this extraordinary book, a testament to the divine intervention of God Almighty and the unwavering love and support of my cherished Family, devoted Fans, avid Readers, loyal Customers, and dear Friends. Their ceaseless encouragement has paved the way for this resounding success.

www.ingramcontent.com/pod-product-compliance
Lightning Source LLC
Chambersburg PA
CBHW031135020426

42333CB00012B/384